know your cat's
Purr Points

D1487921

For my darling mother (1914 - 2000)
who knew all the purr points.

Thorsons
An imprint of HarperCollins Publishers
77-85 Fulham Palace Road,
Hammersmith, London W6 8JB

The Thorsons website address is: www.thorsons.com

First published in Great Britain by Thorsons 2000

10 9 8 7 6 5 4 3 2 1

Text and Illustrations © Margaret Woodhouse 2000

Margaret Woodhouse asserts the moral right to be
identified as the author of this work

A catalogue record of this book is available from the British Library

ISBN 0-00-710724-2

Printed in China

know your cat's
Purr Points

Margaret Woodhouse

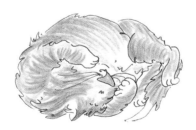

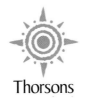

Thorsons

Contents

▲▲▲▲▲▲▲▲

The Pleasuring of Cats

▲▲▲▲▲▲

The giving of pleasure to a cat is an ancient practice. Through the aeons cats have held sway over humans, bewitching them into conducting indulgent acts of pleasuring. Even Stone Age cat gladly accepted attention from its homo sapiens cave-mate.

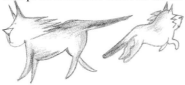

The practice reached its zenith in Ancient Egypt. But only recently have experts appreciated the extent to which the Egyptians considered the pleasuring of a cat such a practical art. While the receipt of pleasure was a most sensual experience for the Subject, the Practitioner approached his task in a manner that was both functional and technical.

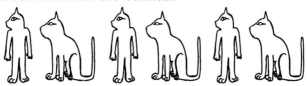

The art of pleasuring cats has never been lost completely. Now, appropriately in this revivalist age, exciting new finds in Egypt have enabled Pleasurecatologists to reconstruct the original Egyptian teachings. These *Purr Points* are reproduced here, ensuring that full prides of happy cats will endure through the millennia.

Indulgent Locations

▲▲▲▲▲▲▲

It is of extreme importance for the Purr Point Practitioner to know exactly in which location to position the Subject when wishing to undertake the pleasuring of a cat.

We recommend the following as excellent choices:

      Best arm chairs (the Ancient Egyptians used thrones)

      Beds (duvets and covers that show the dirt are preferred)

      Kitchen tables

      Wide human laps

      Outdoor sunny locations (flower beds prove
             highly acceptable to the Subject)

Remember, positioning is everything!

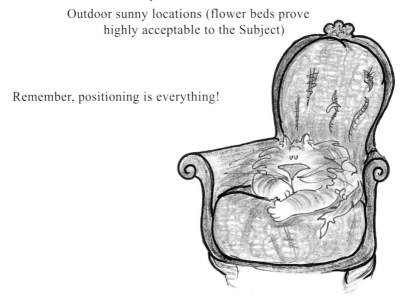

The Pleasuring of the Front

Ancient writings indicate exactly where the critical Purr Points are on a cat. The Practitioner must commit these to memory. Nothing distracts the Subject more than an ill-directed application. (It can also be rather dangerous for the Practitioner.)

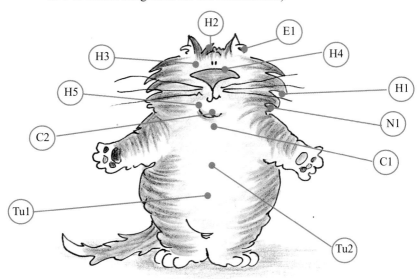

H1	The Inter-whisker Side Step	C1	Chin Lifter
H2	The Rumbler	C2	Ticklers
H3	Knuckle Dusters	Tu1	The Full Fluff
H4	La Petite	Tu2	The Plunge
H5	The Trans-whisker Cross Step	N1	The Flamenco Guitar
E1	Feather Dusters		

The Pleasuring of the Back

▲▲▲▲▲▲▲▲

Note that there are less critical Purr Points for the back. This
reduced sensitivity would appear to result from a failure on the
part of most Subjects to shoulder responsibility.

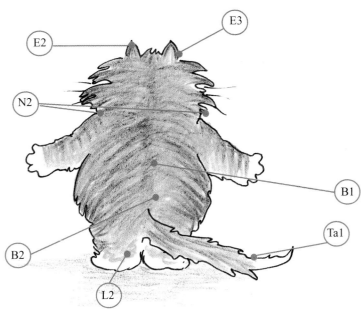

E2	The Flick	B1	Dancing The Limbo
E3	Tipping	B2	Spankers
L2	The Tree Fern	Ta1	Tippers
N2	Double Doser		

The Purr Register

▲▲▲▲▲▲▲

It is not easy to assess the level of pleasure derived by a cat.

For this reason we have developed two pleasure indicators—a modern but excellent addition to the art of Pleasuring the Cat.

Each *Purr Point* is given a rating on both indicators. The Practitioner needs to assess both auditory and visual responses. Thus a rating of only II on the *Purrometer* may be offset by a pose of exquisite response on *The Purr Register*, lifting the overall score to 4.

Purrs are gauged by the *Purrometer*—from I to V. Thus:

I-II "The Mo-ped"
>   Felt only by a few Practitioners, mainly those wearing light apparel.

III "The Harley Davidson"
>   Felt by nearly all Practitioners. Negligible movement by Subject.

IV "The Corvette"
>   Felt by all Practitioners. Some shift in Subject's original position occurs. Fur slightly displaced.

V "The Dump Truck"
>   Felt, even through cushions. Damage through clawing possible. Few if any Practitioners left sitting.

The second of the two pleasure indicators is *The Purr Register*. As some Subjects never purr very much, this highly accurate pleasure ~~assessor allocates a~~ allows a purr level to the non-purrer, judged on looks alone.

1-2　**Pleasant Repose**

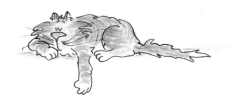

3　**Mild enjoyment**

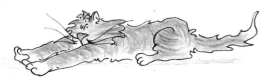

4　**Pleased to be disturbed**

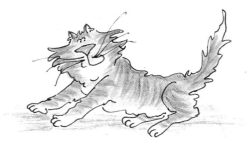

5　**Exquisite response**

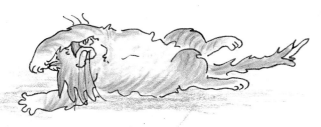

Cautions

▲▲▲▲▲▲▲

Before embarking on any full-scale pleasuring the Practitioner
should first be aware of the following *Claw Points*.

Never surprise the Subject with a
vigorous application. (But see
Spankers p54-55.)

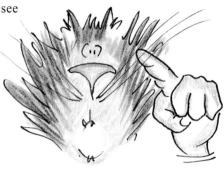

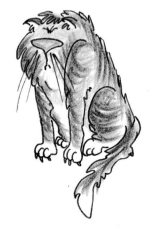

Never attempt an anti-fur-wise
application unless otherwise
instructed.

Should the Practitioner accidentally touch a *Claw Point*, NEVER withdraw the hand at speed.

And remember, enough is almost invariably enough!

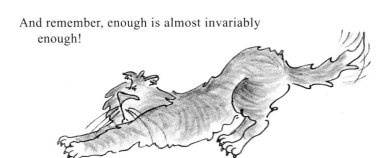

Head Points
▲▲▲▲▲▲

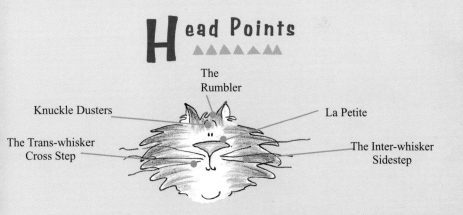

The
Rumbler

Knuckle Dusters

La Petite

The Trans-whisker
Cross Step

The Inter-whisker
Sidestep

When the human polishes the whiskers of a cat
into glittering threads, that is when the lord will
be content to be bound to the slave.

H1 The Inter-whisker Sidestep

▲▲▲▲▲▲▲

👆 Technique

1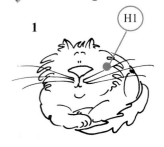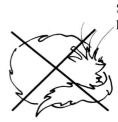

Subject should have head fully accessible.

2

This is a single-full-finger action. Hold hand thus. The aim is to achieve a world-is-at-peace-and-the-dog-is-outside feeling.

3

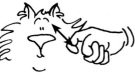

Rub finger rhythmically up and down cheek, and between whiskers until purring is experienced. Moving the finger in a circular motion can also prove effective.

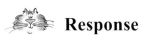 **Response**

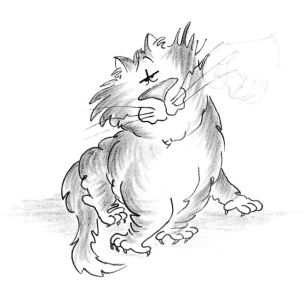

Rating on *The Purr Register*   4

Purrometer reading   V

(Important: Do not prolong the ecstasy unduly. Extended
   application provokes needling on the part of the Subject. This
   can be the cause of great discomfort to the Practitioner.)

(H2) The Rumbler

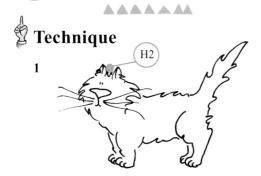

Technique

1

 Many locations will suffice for *The Rumbler*. However, it is difficult to execute if Subject is in full flight.

2

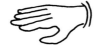 Practitioner's hand is held thus:

3

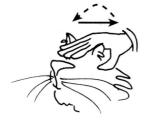 Practitioner moves hand in a fur-wise direction. Be careful to lift hand for each application. (For counter-application, see *Cautions*, pp12-13.)

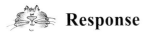 # Response

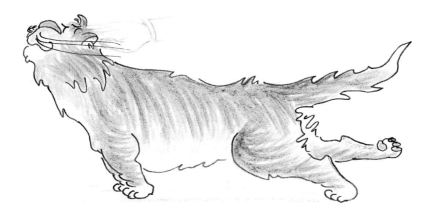

Rating on *The Purr Register*   4

Purrometer reading   III

This is unquestionably the Classic Pleasure. Many applications
   may be conferred every day, and by copious Practitioners.

(H3) Knuckle Dusters

 Technique

1

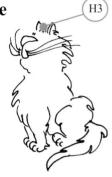

Subject's head must be upright and alert. While it is acceptable to apply the Purr Point while the Subject is standing, the sitting position gives maximum stability.

2

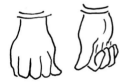

Practitioner's hand should be half-fisted.

3

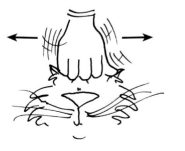

Hold half-fist tautly and, using maximum control, vibrate back and forth with vigour.

Response

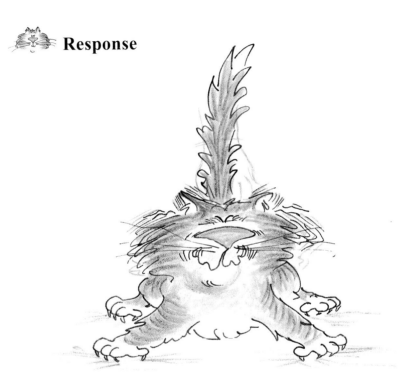

Rating on *The Purr Register* 5

Purrometer reading IV

Knuckle Dusters catches the Subject in an irresistible insist/desist
cycle. (Rough and tumble has always had a respectability in
certain circles.)

(H4) La Petite

▲▲▲▲▲▲▲

✌ Technique

1

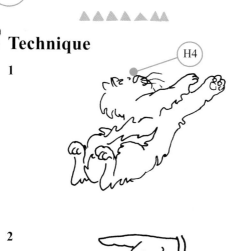

Subject can repose at leisure provided that nose is accessible. Note: This Purr Point is for the bridge of Subject's nose, not the moist health-indicator at the end.*

2

This is a fingertip application. Delicacy is indicated.

3

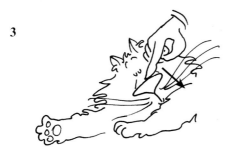

Apply finger to the nose-bridge. Brush rhythmically and slowly in fur-wise direction.

*La Petite is best applied by a Practitioner with an intimate knowledge of the Subject.

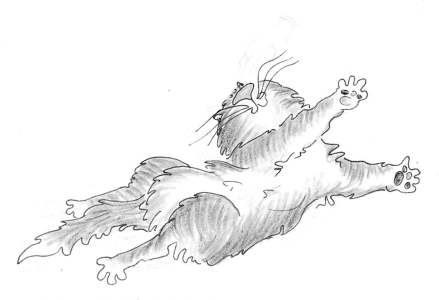

Rating on *The Purr Register*   4

Purrometer reading   II

La Petite engenders a remarkable sense of abandon. Experts
consider this simple application to be the natural prerequisite
for the stimulation of the Tummy Points.

(H5) The Trans-whisker Cross Step

▲▲▲▲▲▲▲▲

✋ Technique

1

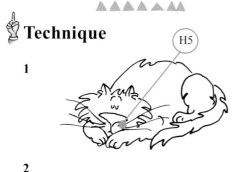

The side of the head must be accessible. Ensure Subject is relaxed.

2

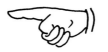

This is a side-of-finger application. Proceed with caution. It is a precarious procedure.*

3

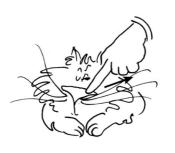

Place finger at edge of Subject's moist health-indicator. Keeping the rest of the hand quite still, move forefinger in a fur-wise direction. Note position of whiskers *behind* finger. (A left-hand application is depicted here.)

*This Application is not for fainthearted Practitioners, nor should it be applied to timorous Subjects.

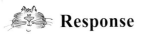

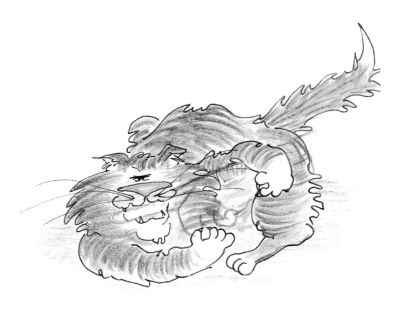

Rating on *The Purr Register* 5

Purrometer reading   0

This is the regrettable result of the misapplication of the *Trans-whisker Cross-step*. (Though it is not to say that the Subject did not derive considerable pleasure from the activity.)

Ear Points

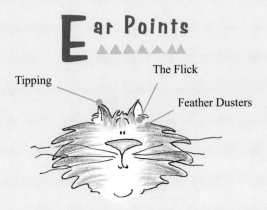

Tipping

The Flick

Feather Dusters

When the Sun God Ra shines upon the ears of a contented cat, all the world will be at leisure and warm thoughts will abound.

(E1) Feather Dusters

☝ Technique

1

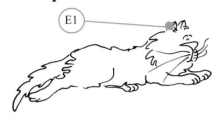

Subject's head should be alert and "in anticipation". The body may repose at leisure.

2

Practitioner's fist in this instance is kept open and fluid, ready for a ripple application.*

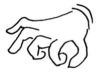

3

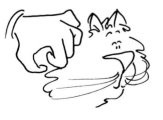

Nestle fist into area at the base of Subject's ear. The second joint of fingers must make a continual rippling while the thumb remains taut and static.

*The success of *Feather Dusters* depends upon a confident delivery.

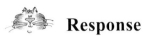 **Response**

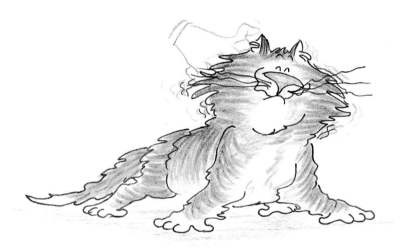

Rating on *The Purr Register* 5

Purrometer reading   V

The effect of the continual rippling is like that of a stone dropped
  into water. The Subject vibrates from the ear outwards. Certain
  Subjects also dribble liberally from the mouth, adding to the
  general aquatic allusion.

E2 The Flick

▲▲▲▲▲▲▲▲

✊ Technique

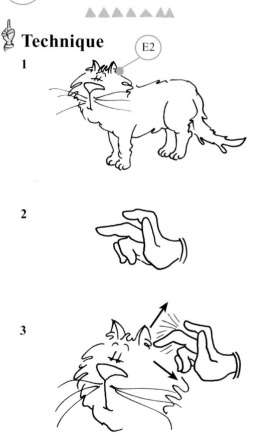

1 Make contact immediately after Subject has been indulging in a languid pastime (eg, a yawn, a milk lap). Subject must be somnambulistic and co-operative.

2 Practitioner's fingers need to work a sharp "re-invigorating" movement.* The middle finger is ideal for this purpose.

3 Apply light staccato taps to lower back of ear. (Note cartilage.) Surprise for *The Flick* is not a disadvantage, unlike most other applications.

The Flick is vital to the Subject's realignment, earthing and general orientation.

Response

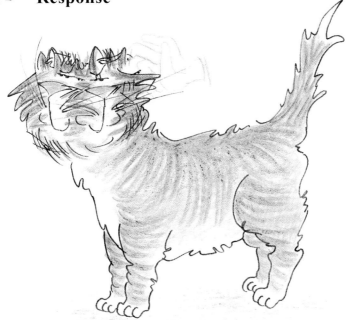

Rating on *The Purr Register*   2

Purrometer reading   I

The Subject will at first display an energised recovery, followed
  by an anti-static manoeuvre (typically, a lightening but
  substantial flick of the Subject's ear).

(E3) Tipping

▲▲▲▲▲▲▲

☝ Technique

1 (E3)

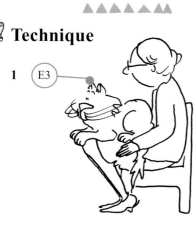

Have Subject sit upon Practitioner's knee, facing outwards.

2

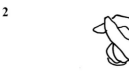

Practitioner will need to work with tips of thumb and forefinger to effect a pincer movement.

3

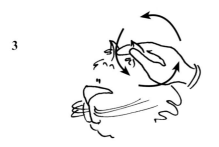

Take tip of Subject's ear between thumb and forefinger, and rub rhythmically in a circular motion.

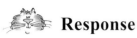 **Response**

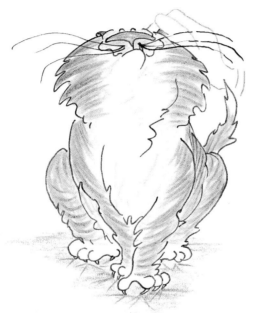

Rating on *The Purr Register* 5

Purrometer reading   V

Carried into a true ecstasy, the Subject will rise to greet the
  application. (Practitioners are advised to wear protective
  clothing.)

Chin & Neck Points

▲▲▲▲▲▲▲▲

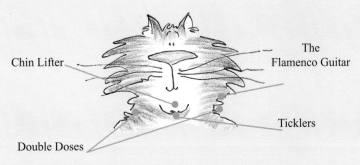

Chin Lifter

The Flamenco Guitar

Ticklers

Double Doses

Behind the jaws of a pussy cat rests the hope and expectations of a lion.

C1 Chin Lifter

▲▲▲▲▲▲▲▲

✊ Technique

1

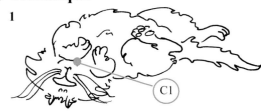

Many positions will prove suitable for application of this Purr Point provided chin is accessible.

2

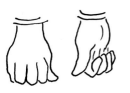

This is a continuous-knuckle application. Practitioner's hands must move with the agility of a pianist warming up for an attack on the keys

3

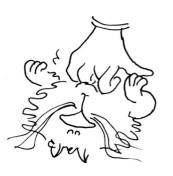

Practitioner gently taps upper chin with forefinger. This activates Subject's anticipation, and lower chin will be lifted. Practitioner then tickles under-chin using the continuous ripple effect.

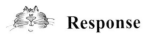 **Response**

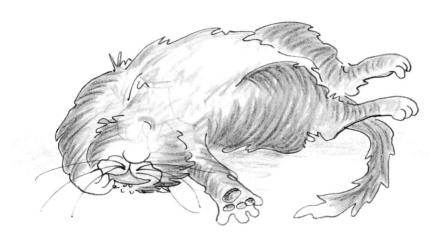

Rating on *The Purr Register*   5

Purrometer reading   V

Somnolence gives way to decadence as the Subject basks in the
   warm glow of the chin-lifter. The Practitioner will be invited to
   even greater excesses as the Subject stretches and extends the
   chin to its uttermost.

(C2) **Ticklers**

▲▲▲▲▲▲

 Technique

1

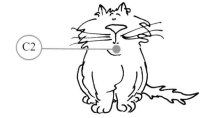

Subject should be in the erect pose.

2

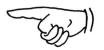

Place forefinger in the "ready" position.

3

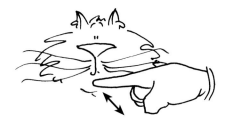

Practitioner approaches Subject from front and application should be administered in rapid fur-wise/anti-fur-wise movements.

Response

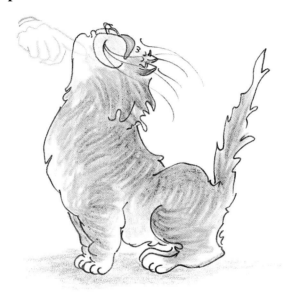

Rating on *The Purr Register*   4

Purrometer reading   V

Ticklers is a glorious celebration of pleasure. The Practitioner will
be tempted to repeat applications by such enticements as full-
throated purring, tail-flicking, and furry vibrating on the part of
the Subject.

N1 The Flamenco Guitar

▲▲▲▲▲▲▲

✊ Technique

1

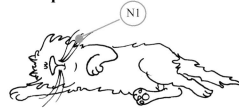

The Subject should be lying in an uncurled position, on the side. The neck should be easily approachable.

2

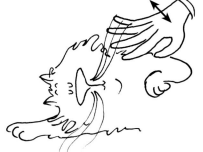

A one-handed application, the Practitioner needs to have fingers taut and extended.

3

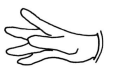

Keeping the fingers rigid at all times, the Practitioner strums the Purr Point with the passion and surprise of a flamenco guitarist.

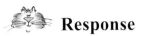 **Response**

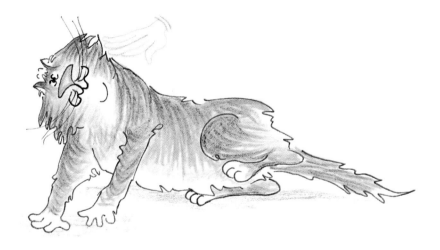

Rating on *The Purr Register*   4

Purrometer reading   II

Most Subjects are disturbed from their torpor by the insistent
Iberian rhythm. Note the low Purrometer reading—an
indication of how preoccupying the strumming can be.

N2 Double Doses

▲▲▲▲▲▲▲

 Technique

1

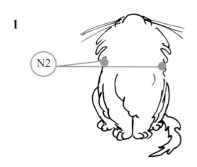

Ideally, apply this Purr Point immediately after application of Purr Point C2. Subject's neck will be perfectly positioned, and desire for further pleasuring will be at its height.

2

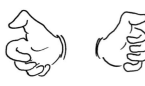

Both hands must be made ready for a continuous-knuckly application.

3

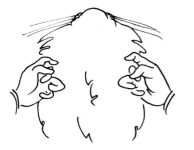

Practitioner approaches Subject from front. Hands must work simultaneously. Take care not to synchronise movements. The syncopation is what provides the thrill.

Response

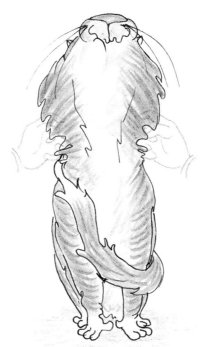

Rating on *The Purr Register* 5

Purrometer reading   IV

The true origin of the expression 'enwraptured' is illustrated in the
   response to this application. Subjects will generally be
   transported into some unrecognisable alter-ego.

Tummy Points

▲▲▲▲▲▲▲

The Full Fluff

The Plunge

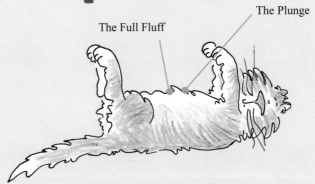

Believe that fur is not simply a convenient barrier worn to keep the cold at bay.

(Tu1) The Full Fluff

▲▲▲▲▲▲▲

✋ Technique

1

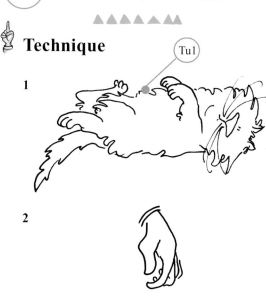

Subject should be in prone position in a location of extreme comfort.

2

Practitioner's hand should be relaxed and feel very malleable.

3

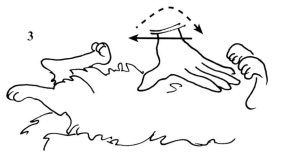

Gently lay hand upon Subject's tummy. Stroke in single fur-wise actions, taking care to lift hand before renewing the stroke.

Response

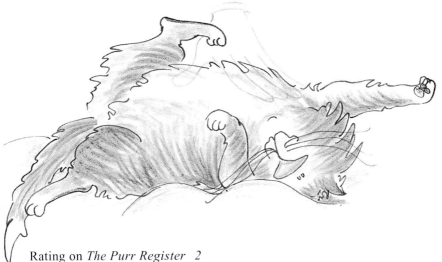

Rating on *The Purr Register*   2

Purrometer reading   V

An application of *The Full Fluff* carries with it a considerable
surprise for the confident Practitioner. Transported, as the
Applicant's hands are, on a bedding of soft fluffy fur, the
purring from the Subject is soon transferred to the Applicant
until both are heard to be throbbing in a happy contentment.

The Plunge

▲▲▲▲▲▲▲

Technique

1

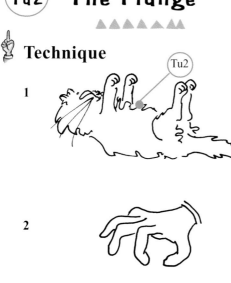

Tu2

Ensure Subject is in prone position.

2

Hold hand thus as for a full-hand assault.

3

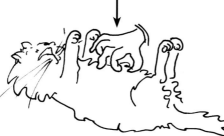

Drop hand on to Subject's tummy and move fingers rapidly and at random.

Response

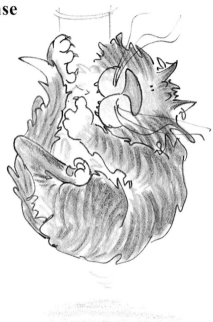

Rating on *The Purr Register* 5

Purrometer reading   IV

The Plunge is a highly dangerous application. However, it is also
a Purr Point from which the Subject will derive considerable
pleasure.

Back & Tail Points

▲▲▲▲▲▲▲

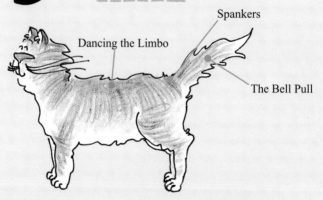

Spankers

Dancing the Limbo

The Bell Pull

Full pleasure does every cat explore with every
back that's arched and every tail that's flicked.

Dancing the Limbo

▲▲▲▲▲▲▲▲

✍ Technique

1

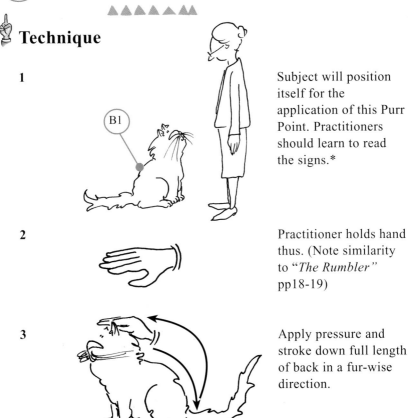

Subject will position itself for the application of this Purr Point. Practitioners should learn to read the signs.*

2

Practitioner holds hand thus. (Note similarity to *"The Rumbler"* pp18-19)

3

Apply pressure and stroke down full length of back in a fur-wise direction.

*If the Subject adopts this position and then commences to "weave", it is more likely to be in preparation for the Ultimate Pleasure. (See p 64.)

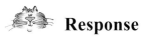 **Response**

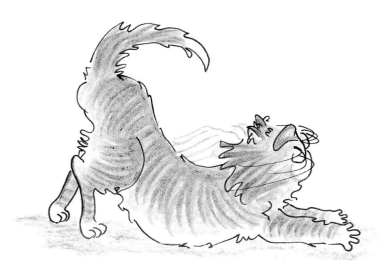

Rating on *The Purr Register* 3

Purrometer reading   II

The most intriguing aspect of this Purr Point is the fact that the
   subject behaves as if avoiding the very pleasure craved.

(B2) Spankers

Technique

1

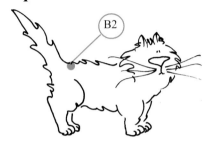

B2

Spankers is one of the few Purr Points best approached with an element of surprise. Subject must be standing.

2

Hold hand out and keep rigid.

3

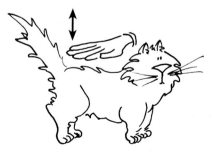

Make firm, rapid patting motions at the precise point of pleasure.

🐱 Response

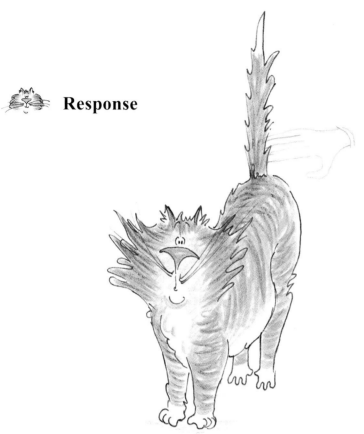

Rating on *The Purr Register* 5

Purrometer reading   0

Despite the *Purrometer* reading, some experts even attribute the
    accolade "The Ultimate Pleasure" to *Spankers*. (Suspect
    proclivities are also referred to in *Knuckle Dusters*, pp20-21.)

(Ta1) # The Bell Pull

▲▲▲▲▲▲▲▲

 Technique

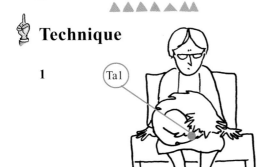

1

Position Subject in indulgent position on Practitioner's lap. Allow to relax totally.

2

Practitioner's hand is held in ready-to-grasp position.

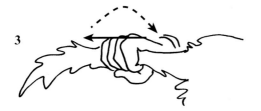

3

Unfold tail from "at ease" position and grasp in fist. Run hand fur-wise down tail. To repeat, release grasp slightly.

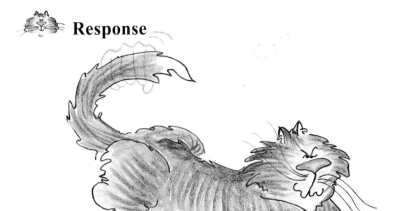

Response

Rating on *The Purr Register*   4

Purrometer reading   IV

Borne into a frenzy of pleasure the Subject will unleash a
   primordial energy causing the Practitioner to "stretch-the-lap".
   This additional muscle manipulation provides exquisite
   secondary pleasure.

Leg Points
▲▲▲▲▲▲▲

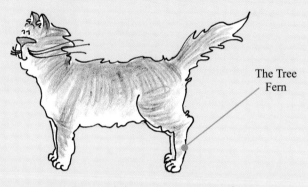

The Tree
Fern

If the legs are fleet and the paws are strong then
the human will be in thrall to a panther.

(L1) The Tree Fern

▲▲▲▲▲▲▲

✍ Technique

1

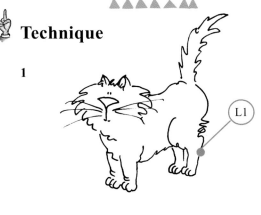

Practitioner is best to approach a standing Subject. The *black stumps* at back of leg must be accessible.

2

Practitioner holds hand thus.

3

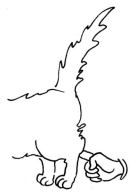

Using inside of forefinger, Practitioner strokes leg stumps downwards. (Note: the fur at this site is generally erect and thus a fur-wise/anti fur-wise direction is difficult to identify.)

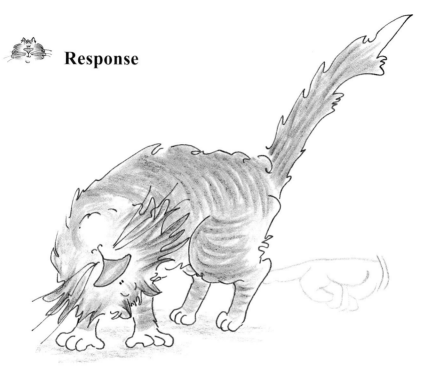

Response

Rating on *The Purr Register* 3

Purrometer reading   II

The Subject will willingly accept the opportunity to contort,
achieving a coy appearance in the process. Practitioners may
well find they contort in the same manner in order to assess the
true level of pleasure being attained.

The Ultimate Pleasure

▲▲▲▲▲▲▲

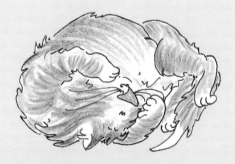

Only when caresses have touched the fur of the cat from one extremity to the other will the full picture of pleasure be truly revealed.

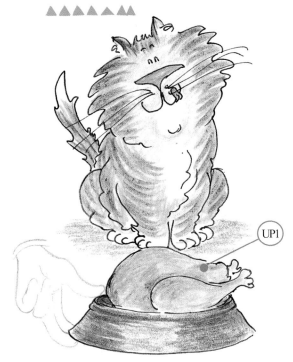

Rating on *The Purr Register*   5

Purrometer reading   V

This Purr Point is named in honour of the circular motion that is
taken by the Subject's tongue when met with the prospect of
this, the Ultimate Pleasure.